RAW FOOD DIET FOR BEGINNERS

Eat Simple and Lose Weight in Easy Way

By

Andrew Low

Table of Contents

4

Raw Food Basics

How To Eat Yourself Healthy

Eating food is simple. But eating simple is one of the most difficult things today. There is not enough natural spring water available to all. And we are not able to digest raw wild green grasses and plants anymore. In addition, there is temptation of cheap junk food everywhere.

Junk food is not natural. Natural alone will endure. Natural eating has endured for thousands of years. Without ever having to spend billions of dollars on marketing. Eating simple and natural is only common sense. An error does not become truth because of repeated advertising. Nor does truth become error because nobody sees it.

What you eat every day expresses your priority. Is your priority to be healthy, energetic and happy? Make the world a better place? Or do you prefer to not having to think or plan, zap TV at home, stay in your comfort zone, and be accepted and liked by others. This is what you have to ask yourself. What is your true priority? Decide and live by it.

Your priority is your goal. To remind yourself daily and motivate yourself to pursue it, write your own goal down a paper and stick it on your fridge, make it your computer password, set an alarm in your calendar to remind you regularly, post an inspiring quote or picture in your bathroom or mirror, read books about the subject, listen to tapes, watch DVDs and go to meetings where the subject of your goal is discussed. Break your goal down in small and easy to do everyday tasks. Then just go.

My priority is being healthy and happy so you can help your family, friends and other interested people to become healthy and happy too. After researching, observing and experiencing, I believe that eating a natural diet is imperative to getting there. To me a natural healthy diet is one that consists of mostly raw, plant based and nutrient dense food.

In this book you will find recipes that are made with these ingredients. Are easy to prepare for starters of a raw food diet and are incredibly delicious. This way it is easy to stay motivated and keep going.

What To Eat

I like to eat food uncooked because when it's raw, it is full of enzymes, easily absorbable minerals and lifo force.

Food is considered raw if it is never heated above 42 C/118 F degrees. In addition, I like it as fresh (and wild) as possible. And of course free of preservative, pesticides, irradiation and genetic manipulation.

Focus on the following food groups:

1. Green leafy vegetables
2. Sea Vegetables (Nori, Kelp, Dulse, Irish Mosh, etc.)
3. (Wild) Herbs & Spices (e.g. Basil, Stevia, Garlic, Cilantro, Ginger, Chili Pepper, Mint)
4. Medicinal Mushrooms (e.g. Shiitake, Maiitake, Reishi, Chaga)
5. Super foods (= food that nutrient dense): e.g. raw chocolate, goji berries, young coconut water, green powders.

6. Wheat grass & Sprouts

7. Seeds (flax, hemp, chia, sesame, pumpkin, sunflower).

8. Food fermented with pro-biotics: e.g. (uncooked) sauerkraut, pickles, beverages, miso.

9. Clean and superb drinking water.

In this book you will find examples on how to use these ingredients to make delicious, satiating and easy to prepare meals. Eating them will boost your energy like you have never experienced before.

Combine these foods with a relaxed lifestyle, happy thoughts and being directly grounded to the earth. Expose your skin and eyes to some direct sunlight every day and miracles might happen.

How To Prepare

You can virtually eat the same on a raw food diet as you would on a cooked diet. What is the most striking difference, besides de ingredients, is the preparation of your food. The following preparation methods are to:

1. Ensure that your food remains below 42 C/118 F degrees
2. Get a preferred consistency
3. Make your food easily absorbable and/or
4. Conserve your food

Preparation Methods

Here are the most used preparation methods for making raw food dish.

1. Juicing
2. Blending
3. Dehydrating
4. Cutting

Juicing

Juicing is a way to get the liquid (juice) out of a vegetable or fruit. The fiber is taken out, the juice is left. This is a way to get concentrated vitamins and minerals that are extremely easy for your body to absorb. The nutrients may enter your blood stream within 20 minutes.

There are three kind of juicers:

1. Citrus juicers (orange juice);
2. Centrifuge juicers (carrots);
3. "Slow" juicers (greens).

Citrus juicers are the ones you use for lemons and oranges. You can buy some hand juicers for about 5 USD. I have cheap glass one I use for quickly juicing lemon juice.

Centrifuge juicers are quick and easy to use. They work well for harder fruits and vegetables such as apples, carrots, cucumber, celery, ginger, beets. You can also use them for whole lemons and oranges (peeled!). You may try to put in some greens, but they don't get much juice out of them. They range in price from 50 - 500 USD. I like the Solis or Breville brand.

Slow Juicers are best used for green leafy vegetables and grasses. But they also work for apples, carrots and cucumbers. They are the most expensive, generally are more work to juice (may have to pre-cut) and to clean. But they are quit and extract the most juice.

Moreover, they generally give you the best quality juice and nutrients because of added magnets and or a gentler way to treat the produce.

Blending

Blending is a way to cut produce so small that it becomes a smooth soup, or "smoothie". High quality high speed blenders such as Blendtec and Vitamix cut the food so tiny that they the cell wall is broken. This makes it easy for you to absorb tough vegetables. Blending uses the whole food, thus the fibre remains.

You can blend fruits, vegetables, greens, super foods, water, nuts, seeds, etc. You can make cold or warm smoothies, sweet or hearty.

Blenders are very easy in use and quick to clean. A very popular way to prepare raw food.

My first raw food year I used a hand blender (700 watt). Relatively inexpensive and it worked really well and I still use one when I travel. Obviously, it doesn't make the food as smooth (especially greens like spinach) and it won't break the cell wall of greens so it is not as easy to absorb the smoothies.

Vitamix and Blendec are the best blenders. They are quite an investment but well worth it because you will use them often.

Dehydrating

Dehydrating is a way to dry your food and take the water out. Once dehydrated, you can store your food in a air tight container or plastic bag. It is also a way to make the food crunchy and often used as an alternative to conventional baking.

Since the food should remain "raw" it cannot be dehydrated in normal oven though. Best ways to dehydrate are to let the food sun dry or use a special dehydrator (i.e. Excalibur). Other ways are to use your radiator or your conventional oven on the lowest temperature.

If you would like to make gourmet food, I would certainly get one. Otherwise, this appliance wouldn't be on top of my list. It's big, expensive and dehydrating at low temperatures takes generally 6 - 24 hours for your food to be ready.

Cutting

You can cut your food with sharp knifes, a cutter, mandoline or food processor.

Sharp knifes are important when preparing raw food and of course a cutting board.

A hand cutter is easy when you need to cut many onions or nuts. Its a bit a hassle to clean them.

A food processor is nice if you want to make a pesto. Thus something not completely smooth (which it will get if you put it in your blender) or for using smaller quantities. I use my hand blender for this and pulse, or use the food processor part of my hand blender. I would only use a food processor for larger quantities. (I generally prepare raw food for just for 1 or 2 people).

A mandoline are for fun. You can make nice shapes, such as potato shapes, ribs, or very thin slices. Relatively inexpensive and nice to have, but not a must.

What Food To Choose

In order to prepare delicious and healthy meals choose the highest quality food. This will hugely impact the success of your dish. Especially, look for organic, fresh and local if you can.

Since you are using fresh products the suggested ingredients in the ingredients list of the recipes may have to be adjusted according to the size or source of the food.

A tip: for this reason, start with only half the amount of the listed ingredients of spices that are spicy or strong such as cayenne pepper or ginger. Taste and then add more if you like. This way you avoid that you will "spoil" your dish with too much ginger or garlic.

Food Safety

When preparing raw food it's important to be hygienic and store your edibles safely.

- Be careful with cutting boards, knifes and plates and wash your hands before preparing and eating your meals.
- Buy only foods from sources you trust.
- Refrigerate your food.
- Don't leave edibles out of the fridge for more than two hours (especially the pate's, nut milks and animal foods).
- You can use food grade hydrogen peroxide to disinfect your food (1 drop is more effective than cooking).
- Don't eat in restaurants, that you don't know and where food isn't prepared before your eyes, hygiene is practiced strictly or where few people come to eat...

The Recipes

The recipes in this book are sorted by when to eat them. Thus breakfast, lunch, dinner, snacks and drinks. (But obviously, you can have a lunch recipe for dinner or vice versa.) Start your morning with a raw food breakfast and work up until all your meals are raw!

Your body will be so grateful that it will get the fuel to heal and clean itself. Animals will thank you because you let them live a good life and the planet will appreciate you eating a raw organic (mostly) plant based diet that will actually regenerate the earth. And Ghandi would have thanked you for "Being the change you want to see in the world".

Thank you for reading this book. I wish you a miraculous increase in health, beauty and happiness.

BREAKFAST

RAW FOOD

RECIPES

Oat Meal

Serves 2

Ingredients

- 2 apples
- 1 banana
- 1 tablespoon golden flax seed
- 2 teaspoons cinnamon purified water

Directions

1. Put the flax seeds in the purified water and let sit overnight.
2. Peel the apples and cut them into small pieces (for the blender).
3. Peel the banana en break in parts. Rinse the flax seeds.
4. Put all ingredients in a blender. This can be a hand blender or high speed blender such as *Vitamix*.
5. Add ¼ cup water, just enough to let the mixture blend well.

6. Blend all ingredients until smooth. You may want to add a little more water if it's too thick.

Tip

- You make this recipe even better by replacing the water with almond cream or fresh juice. You may also add a tablespoon of hemp seeds. My daughter likes to add (germinated) nuts and raisins.

- You can prepare this recipe the night before (but put the banana in there in the morning). Especially with nuts and dried fruits in it, it will only taste better!

Vanilla Yoghurt

Serves 1

Ingredients

- ½ cup coconut water
- 1 cup coconut meat
- ½ teaspoon vanilla extract

Directions

1. Open the coconut with a cleaver.
2. Pour the coconut water in the jar of a high speed blender and some or all of the milk.
3. Blend well. You should get the consistency of yogurt.

Tip

- You can drink it as it is or you can add a fruit of your choice. Think of peach, strawberries, mango or pear. So good!
- A fantastic replacer of yoghurt made from dairy. It's delicious as a yoghurt

desert, for breakfast with granola or you can put it in your ice maker machine and you get delicious ice cream.

Apple Avocado Mousse

Serves 2

Ingredients

- 1 avocado
- 2 apples
- ¼ cup purified water

Directions

1. Peal the apples and take out the core.
2. Take the avocado meat out of the avocado.
3. Put the two ingredients in a bowl. Mix well with a hand mixer.

Energy Bomb Smoothie

This is my favorite raw breakfast recipe. I drink this smoothie every morning, or a variation of it is really good and very filling! A nutritional bomb! Full of minerals, enzymes, co-factors and high quality protein.

I can only use a tiny bit of raw chocolate and I could live on just these smoothies. I drink only 2 a day and then a salad at night. The raw chocolate is a great re- placer for coffee. When you use warm water or tea (not heated above 170 F) you have a nice warm drink.

Ingredients

- 1 teaspoon of raw carob powder (or raw chocolate)
- 1 tablespoon goji berries
- ½ teaspoon maca powder
- 1 teaspoon bee pollen
- 1 tablespoon hemp seed

- 1 teaspoon raw honey (or yucon root or few drops stevia)
- 1 teaspoon green powder (spirulina, chlorella, wheat grass)
- few leafs of greens (such as spinach or dandelion)
- few scoops of coconut meat (optional)
- 2 cups special warm herb tea or pure water or coconut water

Directions

1. Mix all in a blender and enjoy!

Mango Smoothie

This mango smoothie makes a superb breakfast and gives enough energy to last a whole morning. It's raw and vegan. No added sweeteners an dairy free.

Ingredients

- 1 mango
- 2 bananas
- 1-2 oranges
- dash of lemon juice
- 1 tablespoon hemp seed
- ¼ teaspoon green powder
- ice cubes (optional)

Directions

1. Peel and pit the mango, cut into pieces.
2. Peel and cut the banana and orange.
3. Put all ingredients in the blender (orange first). Blend all ingredients well.

Tips

- You may want to add a little water if it's too thick. The hemp seeds provide good fats, super protein and fibers. This smoothie is also delicious with some coconut meat or water (instead of the hemp and orange).

- I often keep frozen mango and/or banana in the fridge. This way I always have the ingredients with me for making this recipe.

Hemp & Berry Smoothie

Serves 2

Ingredients

- 1 Banana
- 2 Tablespoons hulled hemp seed
- 1 Bag of frozen berries
- 1 Cup pure water

Directions

1. Put all ingredients in a high speed blender.
2. Add enough water so that all ingredients are covered. Blend well. You may want to add a little more water if it's too thick. You may blend longer if you find it too cold.

Tip

- The hemp seeds provide good fats and super protein.
- Hemp seeds are the only seeds that have no enzyme inhibitor and therefore

don't have to be soaked in water before eating.

If the berries are sour, you may add a few drops of (liquid) stevia to the smoothie to get a sweeter taste.

LUNCH

RAW FOOD

RECIPES

Guacamole

Serves 3

Ingredients

- 3 avocados, pitted
- 1 onion, diced
- 2 tomatoes, diced
- 2 sprigs fresh cilantro, finely chopped 1 lime or lemon
- 2 gloves garlic cayenne pepper to taste sea salt to taste ½ cup distilled water

Directions

1. Scoop the meat from the avocado skin.
2. Cut the avocados into chunks, place in a large bowl, and mash with a spoon.
3. Gently stir in the onions, tomatoes and cilantro.
4. Squeeze in the lime juice and stir in salt to taste.

Tip

- Absolutely lovely with (self made) flax seed crackers, sprouted bread (i.e. *Ezenkiel)* or the rosemary crackers from *Pure Food & Wine/ 1 lucky duck.*
- Great as a dip for crudités (carrots, celery, broccoli, bell peppers)

Flax Seed Crackers

Serves 4

Ingredients

- 1 cup ground flax seed
- ¼ cup sesame seeds
- ¼ cup buckwheat
- 1 or 2 hand full dried fruit (raisins, goji berries, cut of figs) ½ tablespoon sea salt
- 1 cup water

Directions

1. Mix all dry ingredients in a bowl.
2. Add the water. Mix again.
3. Let stand for at least 2 hours so that the sugar from the fruit can be infused and soaked by the seeds. You may want to stir occasionally to see if there is enough water. It's not absolutely necessary to soak when you used ground flax seeds (as opposed to whole flax seeds) but I find the crackers taste much better if you do.

4. Spread the batter evenly on a tray. I use oven trays with Teflon or silicon sheets, dehydrator trays with Teflon sheets, you can even use a large ceramic plate (but put some coconut oil on the bottom so it will come off easily). You can spread the batter with the back of a spoon, a spatula or with your hands.

5. Now, let's dehydrate. You can do this in a dehydrator, conventional oven at lowest setting and preferably one that can be put on dry air, direct sunlight, on top of a radiator. The key is that the temperature of the food should not be raised above 40 degrees Celsius or 115 Fahrenheit. A food thermometer (used for beef!) may help you determine this.

6. Wait until the top is dried well. In the sun and conventional oven is is about 2 hours. In the dehydrator about 4 hours, depending on how much water was added to the batter.

7. Then flip and let dehydrate for another hour.

Tips

- You can eat the crackers warm or cold. If dried well, you can store the crackers in a container that will keep any moist out. (it's dry when there is no condense in the closed container)
- These crackers is that are great for lunch with avocado, pesto and tomato. You can add any other spread.
- Also great as a snack, or as chips. Just alter this basic recipe.
- What's great about these flax seed recipes with crackers is that the variations are limitless. Experiment with adding other seeds such as hemp seed, or nuts (walnut, brazil, almond).
- Or try adding other dried fruit, such as dates or apricots, even olives or dried tomatoes (cut them in small pieces and let them soak with the seeds). You may want to cut down on the salt if you use olives or dried tomatoes since they are salty by themselves.

- If you make the crackers a little thicker and eat them warm, they truly taste somewhat like bread. (but much better)

Lettuce Wraps

Serves 4

Ingredients

- ⅓ cup hemp seed
- ½ cup lemon juice
- ¼ cup honey or a few drops of stevia (2-3)
- 1 ½ tablespoon chopped ginger
- ½ tablespoon red chili
- 1 tablespoon soy sauce
- 1 cup raw almond butter
- ½ head savoy cabbage, shredded
- 6 very large wild spinach leafs
- 1 carrot
- 1 ripe mango
- 1 handful cilantro leafs
- 1 handful torn basil leafs
- Himalaya sea salt

Directions

1. Cut the carrot into into matchstick-size pieces.

2. Cut the Mango lengthwise into strips, about 1/4 inch (1 cm) thick.
3. In a Vita-Mix or high-speed blender, purée the honey (or stevia), lemon juice, ginger, red chili, and soy sauce.
4. Add the almond butter and blend at low speed to combine. You should get a rather thick consistency. (You may add water if it needs to be thinner)
5. In a bowl, mix the almond butter dressing with the cabbage. The best and easiest way is to do this with you hands or a large wooden spoon.
6. Now you need to roll the cabbage with dressing into a "lettuce" wrap. This is kind of tricky. Place the spinach leaf on a cutting board with the underside facing up.
7. Then you put some of the cabbage mix on the leaf.
8. Add some hemp seeds, a few sticks of carrot, a few pieces of mango, and a few leafs of cilantro and, basil.
9. Try to roll up and the spinach leaf, you might need to stick a cocktail-stick in it

to hold. Do this for all the other spinach leafs until the ingredients are gone.

Tip

- This is my absolute favorite lunch dish. It's an adapted and simplified version of Pure Food & Wine's "Thai Lettuce Wraps". If you ever go to NY, I highly recommend you try them in this restaurant. If you bring this dish to a lunch or potluck, you'll be wowed!
- As an alternative to putting the wraps together yourself, it's actually quite fun to let your guests put the wrap together themselves. This will save you time and it adds to a social special atmosphere of your dinner
- If you live in the US, you can also use collard greens instead of the spinach leafs, but I haven't found them in the Netherlands yet.

Tomato & Olive Salad

Serves 4

Ingredients

- 4 parts cherry tomatoes 1 part olives raw extra virgin olive oil lemon juice to taste
- sea salt and pepper to taste
- handful basil
- arugola or other greens (optional)

Directions

1. Break the tomatoes so that the juice comes out (best in a cup so juice won't spill)
2. Combine the tomatoes and olives in a bowl.
3. Add the olive oil, lemon juice and pepper.
4. Toss.

Just before dinner, add the basil and arugola.

Thai Cole Salad

Serves 4

Ingredients

- ½ cup raw cashews
- ½ cup lemon juice
- 2 tablespoons chopped ginger
- ½ tablespoon red chili
- 1 ½ tablespoon tamari
- 1 cup raw almond or peanut butter
- ½ head white cabbage, shredded
- ¼ cup red cabbage, shredded
- ¼ cup carrots, shredded
- 1 ripe mango, cut in small dices
- 1 handful cilantro leafs
- 1 handful torn basil leafs
- 2 tablespoons of honey (or replace with few drops stevia)
- Himalaya sea salt

Directions

1. Cut the mango into small cubes.
2. Shred the cabbage and carrots.

3. In a high-speed blender, purée the honey, lemon juice, ginger, red chili and tamari.
4. Add the raw almond butter and blend at low speed to combine. To get a thick, cake batter-like consistency.
5. Add water to thin if necessary.
6. In a bowl mix the cabbage and the raw almond butter mixture really well.
7. Add the raw cashews and mango pieces.

Top with leafs of cilantro and basil and a few pieces of mango and or carrots for color.

Avocado Carrot Soup

Serves 2

Ingredients

- 1 Avocado
- 1 Medium carrot
- ¼ Cup almond (hemp or sesame) Milk
- 1 Tablespoon ginger (finely chopped)
- ½ Lemon
- 2-4 Drops liquid stevia or 1 tablespoon of raw honey (optional)
- Pinch cayenne pepper
- Pure Water

Directions

1. Put all ingredients in a high speed blender and mix well.
2. Add some purified water or carrot juice should you like a thicker the consistency.

Tip

- Delicious as dip or soup.

Seaweed Salad

Ingredients

- Seaweed of your choice (raw, unroasted) stevia
- Raw sesame oil
- Sesame seeds
- Tamari lemon juice

Directions

1. For the dressing: combine stevia, oil, soy and lemon juice.
2. Mix with the seaweed.
3. Sprinkle sesame seeds on top

Gazpacho

Serves 4

Ingredients

- 4 tomatoes, diced
- 1 medium white onion, diced
- 2 garlic gloves, peeled and minced
- 3 cups distilled water
- raw apple cider vinegar to taste
- lemon juice to taste
- 1 cucumber, peeled and chopped
- 4 tablespoons freshly chopped cilantro (optional)
- 1 scallion (green part), finely chopped, for garnish
- 1 red bell pepper, seeded, cored, and diced (optional)
- 1 table spoon raw virgin olive oil
- ¼ cup mango, diced in small cubes

Directions

1. Place the tomatoes, onion, garlic, water, vinegar, lemon juice, cucumber and cilantro in a blender and purée.
2. Strain (vegetable press is easiest) to remove any vegetable pieces and pits that are not fully liquefied. (if you have a juicer, you can also put all ingredients in the juicer, using a coarse screen).
3. Chill overnight, if time permits.
4. Before serving, sprinkle the chopped scallions, olive oil, some finely cut cilantro and
5. mango over the top of the gazpacho.

Tip

In stead of red bell pepper, mango and cilantro, you could also use pesto (as a topping).

SALSA AND AFTERNOON BREAK

RAW FOOD

RECIPES

Salsa

Makes about 1 ½ cups

Ingredients

- ½ green bell pepper, seeded, cored and diced 2 tomatoes ½ onion, diced
- 1 garlic clove, chopped
- 2 sprigs fresh cilantro, chopped small
- juice of ¼ lemon
- ¼ cup cold-pressed olive oil
- sea salt, to taste
- chopped jalapeño pepper, to taste

Directions

1. Combine the pepper, tomato, onion, garlic, cilantro, lemon juice and oil in a medium bowl, and toss to fully blend.
2. Season with salt and jalapeño to taste.

Cucumber With Goat Cheese

Ingredients

- 1 English cucumber
- Fresh soft Goat Cheese

Directions

1. Slice the cucumber and spread with goat cheese, hummus or any of the other spreads. (Also great with smoked salmon)

Avocado Cole Slaw

Serves 4

Ingredients

- 1 cup shredded red cabbage
- 1 cup shredded green cabbage
- ½ carrot, shredded
- 1 lemon (juiced)
- 1 garlic cloves, minced
- 1 tablespoon whole grain mustard
- 1 avocado, pitted.
- ½ cup distilled water

Directions

1. Mix the cabbage and carrot together in a large bow.
2. Mix the avocado, mustard, garlic and lemon juice in blender until smooth.
3. Pour the dressing over the salad and toss.

Tip

- You can prepare the cabbage & carrot in large quantity and save in the refrigerator for a few days. Then you'll always have some ready for a quick salad. To prepare, just to add a dressing.

Tapenade

Serves 6-8

Ingredients

- 1 glove garlic
- 1 cup black olives (Natures First Law Italian)
- sea salt & pepper to taste
- olive oil
- juice of 1 lemon to taste

Directions

1. Take the pits out of the olives. (if necessary)
2. Place garlic, olives, olive oil and some juice in a blender and blend. (I prefer not too fine)
3. Add salt & pepper and lemon juice to taste and add some more olive oil to make it nice and smooth.

Pesto

Makes about ¾ cup

Ingredients

- 2 tablespoons pine nuts (soaked 20 min)
- 6 tablespoons extra virgin olive oil
- 3 gloves garlic, chopped
- 6 tablespoons chopped fresh basil
- 1 tablespoon chopped parsley
- pinch sea salt

Directions

1. In a blender, combine all ingredients.
2. Blend until smooth.
3. If the sauce is too thick, add a spoonful of warm water.

Zucchini Hummus

Serves 2

Ingredients

- 1 zucchini, peeled and chopped (about 1 ½ cups)
- 2 tablespoons raw tahini
- ½ lemon juiced
- 1 teaspoon crushed garlic (2 gloves)
- ¼ teaspoon ground cumin
- cayenne pepper to taste
- sea salt to taste

Directions

1. Take the pits out of the olives (if necessary).
2. Place garlic, olives, olive oil and some juice in a blender and blend (I prefer not too fine).
3. Add salt & pepper and lemon juice to taste.

Walnut Pate

Makes about 1 cup

Ingredients

- 1 cup soaked raw walnuts
- 1 tablespoon fresh lemon juice
- 1 teaspoon extra-virgin olive oil
- 1 teaspoon raw soy sauce
- ¼ teaspoon garlic powder
- dash sea salt
- 1 tablespoon minced fresh parsley
- 1 tablespoon minced onion

Directions

1. Place the walnuts, lemon juice, olive oil, soy sauce, garlic powder, and salt in a food processor fitted with S blade and process into a paste. Stop occasionally to scrape down the sides of the bowl with a rubber spatula.
2. Transfer to a small mixing bowl.
3. Stir in the parsley and onion and mix well.

DINNER

RAW FOOD

RECIPES

Pizza

Serves 4-6

Ingredients

For the crust:

- 4 cups walnuts, soaked 1 hour or more
- 4 cups zucchini, grated
- 1/2 cup golden flaxseed, ground
- Salt & pepper, oregano, cayenne pepper to taste

Directions

1. Pulse the walnuts in a food processor or chop into tiny pieces (like couscous), but not completely smooth and transfer the nuts to a large bowl.
2. Add the zucchini, flaxseed, salt and about ¼ cup of water, stirring to combine.
3. Add more water until a sticky dough forms. You may need more or less water.
4. Divide the butter between four 14 –inch *Teflex*-lined dehydrator trays.

5. Using an offset spatula, spread the dough to the edges of the trays. The dough can be a bit gummy and sticky, so it helps to dip the spatula in water as you spread the dough (the excess water will all evaporate in the dehydrator).

6. Dehydrate the flatbread at 115 F for 6-8 hours, or overnight. When the tops are dry, flip them over and peel away the Teflex liners. Dehydrate on screens for another 2-4 hours.

7. Once both sides are dry, slide the flatbread onto a large cutting board.

8. With a large chef's knife, cut into pizza rounds of your preferred size and shape.

9. Place them back on the dehydrator trays and dehydrate another hour or more, as necessary for firm crusts.

Ingredients

For the basis:

- 4 cups hemp seeds
- ½ cup lemon juice

- 2 small cloves garlic
- ¼ cup sesame tahini
- 1 teaspoon sea salt
- 1 cup filtered water

Directions

1. In a food processor, add the nuts, lemon juice, garlic, tahini, and salt.
2. Process, adding water 1/4 cup at a time until you get the smoothie, fluffy consistency of hummus.
3. You may need to add more water, or you may want to add olive oil for a richer hummus – just make sure it has enough stiffness so it will hold the toppings on the pizza without running off the sides of the crust.

Ingredients

For the topping

- 1 pint cherry tomatoes, halved

- 1/4 of large bulb of fennel, shaved very thin on a mandolin 1/2 English cucumber, peeled, seeded, and finely diced 1/2 cup Green Olive Tapenade
- 1/2 cup green olives, pitted and halved

Directions

1. Spread each crust with hummus and top with tomatoes, cucumber, olive tapenade and olives.

Tip

Instead of the hummus and topping described above, you can also spread the crust with raw goat cheese, pesto, tomato, olives, tapenade and/or sun dried tomato tapenade.

Spaghetti Al Pesto Or Marinara

Serves 4-6

Ingredients

- 3 pounds of yellow summer squash/zucchini
- Pesto or marinara sauce:

Topping

- ¼ cup olives, chopped
- ¼ cup tomatoes, chopped
- ¼ cup red bell peppers, chopped ¼ cup red onions, chopped

Directions

1. Thinly slice the yellow squash/zucchini with a sharp knife or mandolin to create strands of "pasta". Set aside.
2. For the pesto/marinara sauce put all ingredients in a blender and blend until creamy.

3. Toss the sauce with the sliced or spiraled squash pasta and serve.

Portobello Mushroom Steak

Serves 2

Ingredients

- 2 Portobello mushroom
- 2 tbsp olive oil
- sea salt and pepper to taste

Directions

1. Wipe off the mushrooms with a paper cloth or mushroom brush (don't use water).
2. Toss all ingredients together in a bowl. Mix well.
3. Let marinate for 5-10 minutes.
4. Put in a dehydrator, (hot air) oven (max 50C/120F degrees), in the sun or on your
5. (heated) radiator for about 1-2 hours or until tender.
6. Eat immediately (great when still warm)

It's that easy! Enjoy.

Tips

- If you serve it warm, it's like having a cooked dish!
- You may serve as it is or you could add some marinated onions, chopped tomato cubes, parsley for decoration.
- Next time try adding raw tamari (gluten free soy sauce), garlic, lemon and or cayenne pepper to the marinade.

Mexican Meat Loaf Recipe For Tortillas

Ingredients

- 1 cup walnuts - soaked for 2 hours
- 1 cup sun dried tomatoes - soaked for 1 hour
- Mexican herb mixture (ground cumin, cayenne pepper)
- 1 inch chili pepper (remove the seeds if you don't like it too spicy)
- 1 ripe tomato
- olive oil
- 1 teaspoon tamari
- 2 drops stevia (or 1 tbsp honey, maple syrup)
- handful fresh cilantro leafs

Directions

1. Put all ingredients except tomato, onions and cilantro in a food processor and mix well.

2. Cut onions, tomato and cilantro in small pieces

3. Put all ingredients in a bowl. Mix with a fork until well combined.

4. Test for seasoning. Since the dried tomatoes are usually quite salty, I often don't add extra salt. But taste before adding extra salt to make sure.

Tips

- Great with guacamole and salsa, and tortillas for a real Mexican meal.
- If you change the seasoning and leave out the Mexican herb mixture but add pepper, you can make small meat balls.
- Great with the pasta marinara.

Tortillas

Ingredients

- 1 cup ground flax seed
- 1 cup sweet corn (fresh from cob or refrozen) ½ teaspoon sea salt
- 1 cup spring water

Directions

1. Put the corn in a high speed blender or food processor and mix well.
2. Add to bowl with other ingredients.
3. Mix all ingredients well with a fork, spatula (or hand)
4. Spread thinly onto *teflex* sheets or baking paper and put on baking or dehydration tray.
5. Dehydrate at 115° F or 40° C in dehydrator, hot air oven or in direct sunlight for about 4-6 hours.

Tip

Great with guacamole or salsa!

Raw French Fries Recipe

Serves 4

Ingredients

- Fries
- 4 kohlrabi's
- ½ cups cold pressed olive or hemp seed oil
  2 teaspoons curcumin (kurkuma)
- 1 teaspoon sea salt

Directions

1. Cut the kohlrabi's like french fries (julienne). You cando this with a knife, but it's easiest with a mandolin. There are also special fries cutters you could buy if you think you'll make this a lot.
2. Put the kohlrabi's in a bowl.
3. Put the oil, curcumin and salt in a bowl.
4. Mix and pour over the fries.
5. Let sit for at least 10 min. Then drain and scoop onto some paper towels (to take off excess oil).

Ketchup

- 3 tomatoes
- 3 pieces sun dried tomatoes
- 5 dates (or ½ teaspoon stevia and
- 4 more sun dried tomatoes)
- 1 squeeze lemon juice
- ½ cup pure water

Tip

- Put all ingredients in a blender. On thebottom of the blender the water, lemon juice and tomatoes, on top the dried tomatoes and dates.
- Blend well. This will be easier if you leave the sun dried tomatoes sit in water for a few hours.

Raw Broccoli Salad

Serves 8

Ingredients

- ¼ pound broccoli
- 1 bunch scallions (green parts only) finely chopped (optional)
- 1 cup raw slivered almonds
- 1 cup raw germinated hemp seed
- Dressing:
- 1 cup sesame oil
- juice of 1 lemon
- 1 glove of minced garlic
- 1 small peace of minced ginger
- ¼ teaspoon stevia (o 2 tablespoons honey)
- 1 tbl spoon of tamari (optional)

Directions

1. Slice the broccoli into thin strips as you would cabbage for cole slaw.

2. Toss the broccoli, scallions, slivered almonds and hemp seeds together in a large bowl and set aside.
3. To make the dressing, put the all ingredients in a blender and blend briefly.
4. Pour the dressing over the salad and toss to combine.

Waldorf Salad

My mother makes the best Waldorf salad. Here's the raw and vegan version (replaces chicken, potato and mayonnaise).

serves 2-4

Ingredients

- 2 stalks celery (cut in tiny cubes)
- ½ cup walnuts (soaked for about 2 hours), cut in quarts 3 apples, cut in small cubes
- 2 avocados, cut in large cubes
- 1 grapefruit, peeled and completely stripped of all tiny skins and white pieces.
- kohlrabi or jicama, in small cubes
- salt & pepper to taste

Directions

1. Put al ingredients except 1 avocado in a bowl and mix until well combined.
2. Let stand for about 30 minutes.
3. Add the cubes of the second avocado.

4. Serve immediately.

5. Garnish with parsley, pieces of grapefruit, tomatoes and/or lettuce.

Tips

- If you're not completely raw, you may want to add artichoke harts (cooked).
- I usually serve all ingredients in separate bowls. Then all family members can make their own salad and choose what they like. The kids love it this way.
- You can even add some non raw ingredients such as the artichoke harts for "cooked" members/guests.

Lasagna

serves 2-3

Ingredients

- 2 medium zucchinis
- 2 tablespoons olive oil
- pinch sea salt
- 3 ripe tomatoes
- fresh basil, cilantro and/or spinach leafs.

Direction

1. Using a mandolin, cheese slicer or veggie peeler cut long strips of zucchini (as if you would put them on a grill).
2. Put all zucchini strips in a bowl and add olive oil and salt and mix.
3. Let stand to marinate for about 30 minutes. This will soften the zucchini.
4. In the mean time, prepare the ketchup and vegan cheese. Make about ½-1 cup of each.
5. Cut the tomatoes in slices.

6. Now, take out the zucchini and put on a paper towel to drain any excessive oil or liquid.

7. In a glass or ceramic square bowl (like one you'd use for making lasagna) line the bottom with a layer of zucchini. They should overlap each other slightly so that you can scoop them out without your lasagna falling apart.

8. Then add a layer of ketchup, some slices of tomato and basil, cilantro or spinach leafs.

9. Add a thin layer or a few dots of vegan cheese.

10. Again add a layer of zucchini, ketchup, tomato, green leafs, vegan cheese.

11. Repeat one more time. Thus total of 3 layers.

Fruit Pizza

A children's favorite. Especially if you let them decorate the pizza.

serves 4

Ingredients

Crust

- 2 cups almond flour
- 2 tablespoons agave, maple syrup or honey, 4 drops liquid
- stevia (or to taste)
- pinch sea salt
- ⅓ cup coconut butter
- 2 Cups *Vanilla Cream* (see cookies, cake and desserts)
- Fresh fruit selection (such as bananas, kiwis, blueberries, strawberries, pineapple, pear, raspberries, etc.)

Directions

1. Put al ingredients in a bowl and mix until well combined.

2. Make a ball.

3. Flatten the ball on your plate until it's nice and round like a small pizza. (You may want to put a piece of baking paper or coconut oil on your plate first to make sure you can peel off the "pizza crush" easily)

4. Add a layer of vanilla cream.

5. Decorate with the sliced fresh fruit. You can make faces or art of all kinds!

Tips

- A really fun activity for kids.
- A most delicious dessert!
- If you're hard core raw foodist or lover of tropical fruits, you may replace the vanilla cream with cream of durian (a tropical fruit). It's my very favorite fruit and you can put the meat in a blender to make cream. To me this is true custard. But be warned. The smell of it is pretty strong and is not appreciated by all (or should I say "most"). So I recommend it only if you can prepare/serve the pizza outside and when

you know, only people that love durian will be joining you for the pizza!

For a quick crust you can also use the energy bar recipe.

COOKIES, CAKE AND DESSERT

RAW FOOD

RECIPES

Energy Bars

Serving: About 6 bars

Ingredients

- 1 ½ cups dates (or mix)
- 1 cup nuts (i.e. raw cashews, almonds, pecans, or mix) pinch of salt

Directions

1. Pit the dates and place into a bowl.
2. Turn the dates into a paste. I use a knife and cut them in small pieces. If you do it in a blender or food processor, the dates stick to the knifes.
3. Place the nuts in a food processor, hand slicer or do it by hand with a sharp knife or cleaver. Process them but don't blend to a powder. The bars taste better with tiny pieces of nuts in them.
4. Add the nuts to the dates and mix. This is easiest with your hands. Mix until fully combined.

5. Take the doughy and make 2 long "snakes".
6. Flatten the top and edges with a wooden spoon.
7. Cut each "square snake" into 3-4 pieces. You may wrap each one in baking paper (or plastic wrap). You can even put stickers on the wrap or draw on the paper to really surprise yourself, partner or kids.
8. Store them in the fridge until ready to eat. They travel well, are a great afternoon snack and make happy kids if you put them in their lunch box.

Tips

- This is just the basic recipe. Your variations are limitless.
- Mix dates with figs, apricots, dried apple, raisins, goji berries or try a different combination of nuts.
- It's also delicious with hemp seed or sesame seeds. Just make sure the proportions are bout 1 1/2 fruit and 1 nuts.

- Add vanilla, cinnamon, chocolate powder or lemon juice for extra delicious taste.
- If you find making bars and wrapping them too much hassle. You can also just roll balls.

Dark Chocolate Sauce

Ingredients

- 4 heaped tablespoons of chocolate powder
- 3 tablespoons of raw agave nectar
- ½ teaspoon of coconut oil

Directions

1. Mix all ingredients together to form a paste. If you need it runnier, add more agave nectar.
2. If you need it creamier, add more coconut oil.
3. Wonderful on top of raw ice-cream!

Tip

- Fantastic topping for ice cream or fresh fruit (strawberry) bowls.

Raw Chocolate Cake

Serves 10

Ingredients

- ½ cup cocoa powder
- ½ cup carob
- ½ cup finely ground almonds ⅓ cup agave syrup
- ¼ cup coconut or cacao butter Pinch of sea salt
- For the chocolate filling
- 2 cups cocoa powder
- 1 ½ cups agave syrup
- 1 cup coconut or cacao butter
- 1 tablespoon Vanilla extract (optional)
- 1 tablespoon Lucuma Powder (optional)
- 1 teaspoon Maca Powder (optional)
- For garnishing: strawberries, raspberries, or oranges

Directions

Crust

1. Combine and mix all ingredients. You can best do this by hand or standing mixer). It should have a dough-like consistency.
2. Press the dough evenly into a 7 inch tart pan. (A removable bottom, a plastic cling wrap lining or one of these new flexible silicon pans are easiest.)
3. Chill in the fridge for at least an hour if you have time.

Filling

1. Blend all the ingredients in a blender until very smooth.
2. Poor into the cake crust.
3. Put the cake back in the fridge and chill for at least another hour.
4. Before serving, decorate the cake with the berries, orange or other nice looking fruit.

Chocolate Delight

Serve 4

Ingredients

- meat of 2 young coconuts
- water of 1 young coconut (place the water of 2nd coconut to the side)
- ¼ cup raw cacao powder
- 4 tbl raw Yacon powder
- 4 tbl raw Lacuma powder
- 4 tbl Irish Moss
- 1 tbl raw vanilla bean powder
- 1 tsp cinnamon
- pinch sea salt
- Stevia Liquid extract to taste
- organic quartered strawberries
- organic mint leafs

Directions

1. Place coconut meat and first portion of coconut water in Vita-Mix.

2. Add the rest of the ingredients and with plunger begin to blend.
3. Slowly add water of second coconut to bring to creamy consistency... blend until smooth with texture of a crème.
4. Serve in your favorite glass and garnish with strawberries & mint leafs.
5. Let chill in fridge for 20-30 minutes and enjoy!

Tips

You can use this recipe to make a parfait:

- Separately blend meat of two young coconuts adding coconut water slowly getting a smooth creamy texture.
- Add ground vanilla bean powder.
- 1st Layer Chocolate Crème
- 2nd Layer Vanilla Coconut Crème,
- 3rd Layer quartered organic strawberries, and begin again with Chocolate Crème until glass is filled to the brim!

Garnish, chill, and enjoy!

Blueberry Pie

Serves about 10

Ingredients

Crust

- 1 ½ cups coarse almond flour
- 1 ½ cups fine almond flour
- 3 dates
- ¾ cup raw honey or maple syrup ¾ cup coconut butter large pinch of sea salt

Filling

1. 1 cup raw cashews, soaked for 2 hours or more 1 cup coconut meat ⅓ cup agave nectar
2. ¼–½ cup distilled water at room temperature 6 tablespoons coconut butter
3. 1 tablespoon plus 1 teaspoon almond extract
4. seeds from ½ vanilla bean, or 2 teaspoons vanilla extract pinch of sea salt 6 cups blueberries

Directions

1. In a medium bowl, mix together all the crust ingredients, until very thoroughly combined. Line individual tart shells with squares of plastic wrap.

2. Divide the dough between the shells and press evenly into the sides and bottom, to create an even thickness throughout.

3. Refrigerate until firm, about 1 hour or more and keep refrigerated until ready to fill.

4. In a high-speed blender, purée all the cream ingredients until completely smooth, stopping to scrape the sides as necessary. You may use a spatula to push the mix down into the blades for easier blending.

5. Add more coconut water to thin, but avoid adding too much or the cream will not stay as firm in the tart shells.

6. Fill each tart crust with the cream, creating a flat surface at the top, cover and return to the refrigerator to chill and set about 2 hours or more.

7. For the serving: Remove the tarts from the refrigerator and use the overhanging edges of the plastic wrap to carefully pull the tars from the shells (or push from the bottom if using shells with removable bottoms).

8. Arrange the blueberries on top of each and serve.

Macaroons

Makes 24 to 36 macaroons

Ingredients

- 3 cups dried, unsweetened coconut flakes
- 1 ½ cups raw cocoa powder (or carob powder) 1 cup maple syrup or raw honey ⅓ cup coconut butter
- 1 tablespoon vanilla extract
- ½ teaspoon sea salt

Directions

1. In a large bowl, combine all the ingredients and stir well to combine. You can also use a standing mixer with the paddle attachment.
2. Using a big tablespoon, spoon rounds of the dough onto the dehydrator screens.
3. Dehydrate at 115 F for 12-24 hours, or until crisp on the outside and nice and chewy on the inside

Tips

For blonde macaroons, replace the cocoa powder in the recipe above with an equal amount of fine almond flour.

Apple Pie

Ingredients

Crust

- ¾ cup almonds, soaked overnight (8-12 hrs) 1 ½ cup date pieces or chopped dates
- ½ vanilla essence
- dash cinnamon
- 2 teaspoons psyllium or flax seeds

Filling

- 10-12 apples (peeled and cored), cut in chunks 2 cups dates(pitted)
- 1 cup raisins
- 1 tablespoon of lemon juice
- 2 teaspoons cinnamon
- 2 table spoon psyllium or flax seed

Directions

Crust

1. After draining the almonds, dry them with a wet towel.
2. In a food processor, chop the nuts until they're evenly ground.
3. Add the dates and process until they are finely ground.
4. Then add vanilla and cinnamon while processing.
5. The crust must appear slightly damp and must hold together before adding the psyllium or flax. Add a small amount of water, if necessary.
6. Gradually add the psyllium/flax seeds. Immediately press the mixture into a 9 inch (22,5 cm) pie pan.
7. Dehydrate the crust for 1 hour or leave it in the sun for 1-2 hrs or in a warm oven for 20 min. or use the crust immediately.

Directions

Filling

1. In a heavy-duty juicer, using a blank screen, alternate putting the apples, dates

and raisins through the machine and into a bowl.

2. There should be at least 6 cups of apple sauce mixture, if not, a more apples and put the mixture through the juicer again. For best results transfer the mixture to a food processor and process until very smooth.

3. Add cinnamon, process until mixed.

4. With the processor running, gradually sprinkle in the psyllium/flax seed. Process until thoroughly mixed.

5. Immediately pour the filling into the pie crust, cover and refrigerate.

6. Top with thinly sliced apples that have been dipped in lemon juice.

7.

Ice Cream

serves 4

Ingredients

- 1 cup coconut meat
- 1 cup cashew nuts
- 1 teaspoon stevia (or ½ cup agave syrup or honey)
- 1 teaspoon vanilla powder or 1 vanilla bean
- dash sea salt

Directions

1. Put all ingredients in a blender and blend until completely smooth.
2. Process through your ice-cream maker according to instructions (is quicker if you first cool in fridge)

Tips

This is the basis ice-cream recipe. Your variations are limitless:

1. Add fruit of your choice such as strawberries, mango, banana, pear, blueberries.
2. Add lemon juice or raw cacao powder - and add more stevia to the recipe.
3. If you can't find coconut, you may also replace the coconut and cashews with 2 cups fresh almond milk (or other nut milk)

Vanilla Cream

Serves 3-4

Ingredients

- 2 Cups Coconut Meat
- 1 Cup Cashew Nuts (optional)
- ½ cup Coconut water
- 1 teaspoon ½ cup agave syrup
- 1 teaspoon vanilla powder or 1 vanilla bean

Directions

1. Put all ingredients in a blender and blend until completely smooth.

Tip

This cream makes a great desert with fresh fruit or as is. You may also run it in your ice cream maker for a delicious creamy ice cream.

SMOOTHIE, MILKS AND JUICES

RAW FOOD

RECIPES

Carrot Juice

Ingredients

- 1 lbs large carrots (washed and peeled)
- ½ lemon (peeled)
- few green leafs such as red lettuce or carrot greens 1 apple

Directions

1. Put all ingredients in your juicer. (a centrifuge juicer is easiest for carrots.)
2. Mix and drink immediately.

Tips

- I peel the carrot for taste (otherwise it tastes too earthy). I find this recipe sweet enough, but if you're a beginner juicer or have a sweet tooth, add an apple for extra sweetness.
- The health benefits of carrot juice? It provides Vitamin A, B Vitamins, Vitamin E and many minerals (including calcium).

- Great for pregnant and nursing mothers, eyesight, bones and teeth, liver and nails, skin and hair as well as helping in breast and skin cancer prevent.

Spinach Vegetable Juice

This juice recipe is perfect for starters of veggie juicing. It's soft and sweet. Very tasty. Not bitter or strong at all.

Ingredients

- 1 bunch spinach
- 2 apples
- ½ lemon, peeled (optional)

Directions

Put all ingredients in your juicer. A twin gear juicer such as the Green Star Juicer or slow juicer is best for extracting greens.

Tomato Vegetable Juice

Are you looking for the best of all tomato juice recipes! This one is!

You can juice the tomatoes in a juicer but if you have a high speed blender - such as a *Vitamix* or *Blendec* Blender - and you like more "body" to your juice, you might like to usethe blender in stead.

Ingredients

- 3 cups chopped tomatoes
- 1 stalk celery
- 1 cucumber
- 3 drops stevia (optional)
- ½ teaspoon himalaya sea salt pepper
- cayenne pepper

Directions

1. Juice the tomatoes, celery, cucumber in your juicer.

2. Add drops stevia if you like a sweeter taste, salt, pepper and cayenne pepper to taste.

If you like you can also add a ¼ onion, fresh oregano and basil and red bell pepper.

Cabbage Vegetable Juice

Cabbage juice is known for its ability to heal peptic ulcers. It is full of vitamin K, C, fiber, manganese, B6, Folic Acid, Omega 3 fatty acids, calcium, phytonutrients and anti-oxidants, and very low in calories.

Ingredients

- 1 Head cabbage (red or green)
- 2 Apples or large carrots
- 1 Lemon, peeled

Directions

1. Take off the outer leafs.
2. Cut the head in pieces small enough to fit through your juicer
3. Run through your juicer.

Tips

- **Cabbage is good for you**! Recent studies show that people who eat most cabbagehave a significantly lower risk of colon, lung, breast and prostate cancer. Even compared to other people that eat lots of veggies.

- Red cabbage has even more nutrients and protects against Alzheimer's disease. Juicing cabbage is a superb way to get the best out of your cabbage.

- Cabbage provides anti-carcinogenic glucosinolates (anti cancer fighters).

- When you cook cabbage, you kill the special myrosinase enzyme that makes the cabbage so healing, thus making cabbage less effective as anti cancer food.

- Drinking it straight might be a little too much in the beginning. Then, simply mix it with carrot juice. Start with juicing carrots. Every day add some cabbage leafs until you're used to the taste. (the taste isn't that strong).

- You may also try other cruciferous family members of cabbage such as kale, broccoli, and collard greens.

Kale Banana Smoothie

Ingredients

- 2 bananas
- 2 tablespoons hulled hemp seed
- 1 bag frozen blue berries
- 2$\frac{1}{2}$ cups pure water
- 1 teaspoon super foods of choice (optional)
- 5 leafs kale

Directions

1. Put all ingredients in a high speed blender.
2. Add enough water so that all ingredients are covered.
3. Blend well.

Tips

- Add a little more water if you like your smoothie thinner.
- This is a great way to add (wild edible greens) to your raw food diet. You won't even notice it. This smoothie is full of

important minerals, vitamins, healthy omega three fats, fiber, protein, enzymes, that is hydrating and easy to digest!

Dandelion Apple Smoothie

This yummy recipes is another favorite of mine. It's great with spinach too. Just replace the dandelion with spinach.

Ingredients

- 1 bunch dandelion greens 1 lemon (peeled)
- 2 large apples
- 1 banana
- 2 teaspoons flax seeds (optional)
- Spring or distilled water

Directions

1. Put all ingredients in the blender.
2. Add enough pure water so all ingredients are covered.
3. You can add a banana for creaminess (optional).
4. Blend well and drink.

Arugula Lettuce Pear Smoothie

Ingredients

- 1 banana
- 2-3 pears
- 2 tablespoons hulled hemp seed
- 1 bag of frozen raspberries
- 2½ cups pure water
- 1 teaspoon super foods of choice
- small bunch arugula lettuce
- liquid stevia to taste

Directions

1. Put all ingredients in a high speed blender.
2. Add enough water so that all ingredients are covered. Blend well.

Tip

- Arugula lettuce and pear are an excellent combination. Very delicious and nutritious smoothie.

- You might try this combination in a salad too.

Carrot Ginger Smoothie

Ingredients

- 1 bunch of carrots with some of its greens
  1 avocado ½ lemon
- ⅓ inch fresh ginger, finely cut (like cloves)
- pinch of sea salt and cayenne pepper
- spring or distilled water

Directions

1. Put all ingredients in your juicer.
2. Add clean water to cover all ingredients.
3. Blend and enjoy immediately.

Green Smoothie

The best green smoothie recipe is the one you make yourself. It's very easy and the options are endless. Just have a ration of about 50% fruits and 50% vegetables (or try some wild greens such as nettles) and your smoothie will always be delicious. If not sweet enough, add some liquid. You'll hardly taste the vegetables.

Ingredients

- 1 bunch green leafy vegetable of choice (50% of total) Fruit of choice (50% of total)
- 1-2 Bananas or 1 avocado to emulsify (make creamy) ginger, lemon, parsley or stevia to taste

Directions

1. Put all ingredients in your blender.
2. Add clean water to cover all ingredients.
3. Blend.

4. Drink immediately.

Almond Milk

Ingredients

- 2 cups (spring) water
- ½ cup raw almonds
- pinch of salt
- few drops or half stick vanilla (optional) few drops stevia to taste (optional) nut milk bag or cheese cloth

Directions

1. Let almonds soak overnight in water(for better digestion).
2. In the morning rinse and drain the almonds.
3. Then put them in your blender or jar. Add 2 - 3 cups of clean (spring) water and a pinch of salt.
4. Blend well.
5. Poor the almond milk in the nut bag. It's easiest if you have a large bowl underneath to catch the filtered milk.

6. Now holding the bag with one hand, squeeze the milk with your other hand (see the video of Victoria Boutenko on the website).
7. Add the other (optional) ingredients and blend briefly if needed.

Tips

- If you dehydrate the almond pulp you can use it to make raw cakes and cookies.
- Drink the milk as is or use in smoothies, soups or other recipes. Many friends save it in the fridge for about 2 days (shake before drinking), although I prefer to drink it fresh.
- You can buy nut bags at most health stores and online. They're about 5 dollars each. You can also use nylons, cheese cloth or paint strainer.

Going to the store to buy soy, rice, nut or cows milk takes a whole lot longer and is much more expensive than making fresh almond milk. A *Vitamix* (or any other blender) full with fresh almond milk costs you about 50 cents. You make the almond milk less than 10 minutes.

Hot Chocolate

Serves 1

Ingredients

- 1 cup *almond milk* made with warm water (up to 115 F or 45 C)
- 4 tablespoons raw chocolate powder
- 1 tablespoon honey or coconut nectar
- liquid stevia to taste

Directions

1. Blend the raw chocolate powder and honey/coconut nectar into a paste.
2. Add the almond milk and blend well. Serve immediately.

Tip

- For hotter chocolate, make the almond milk with half the amount of water. Blend all the ingredients, then add 2 cups hot water. Whisk and serve.

Alkalize For Health

How alkaline your blood is, is an easy way to measure the level of your health. A healthy person has a blood pH of 7.365. Generally, a person who is terminal ill has a pH of around 5 or lower.

What Are Alkaline, Acid And PH?

Alkaline foods are foods that raise the the amount of oxygen that your blood takesin. The most alkalizing foods are RAW green leafy vegetables, non-sweet fruits and (wheat) grasses. The opposite of alkaline foods are *acid foods*.

How much oxygen your blood can absorb is measured on a **pH scale** that ranges from 0 to 14. A pH of 0 is most acidic while a pH of 14 is most alkaline.

Alkaline Foods List

During most of your lives, the majority of the foods you eat are (highly) acidic. These make you sick and tired. By eating raw alkaline foods and drinks, you can help your body to heal itself from many chronic diseases.

As a general rule the following foods groups are alkalizing:

- Green leafy vegetables (e.g. spinach, kale);
- Wild greens (e.g., dandelion, nettles, wild grasses);
- Fresh herbs (e.g. parsley, cilantro, basil, garlic);
- Grasses (e.g. wheat, barley grass);
- Sprouts;
- Sea vegetables (e.g. kelp, nori, dulse, spirulina, blue green algae);
- Medicinal mushrooms (e.g. shiitake, maitake, reishi).

Acid Foods List

It's too bad that *the foods you may like most* make you most acidic and thus sick:

- Junk & Processed foods;
- Sugar;
- All animal food (meat, eggs, chicken, fish, lobster, oysters);
- Grains: (white) wheat, rice, pasta, flour, bread etc.;
- Some Fruits;
- Dairy products (milk, cheese, butter);
- Bad fats;
- Peanuts, cashews.

The **best alkaline drinks** are alkaline water, young coconut water, vegetable juice and wheatgrass juice. If your very acidic you might need alkaline supplements to get you back in balance quicker.

How Healthy Are You?

How do you know your body pH? You simply buy some pH test strips (also called litmus paper) at a health store and pee on one. The paper will tell you instantly what your pH is and thus, how alkaline or acid you are (and how healthy).

What Is The PH Scale

PH stands for **P**otential for freeing **H**ydrogen ions. The difference between acidity and alkalinity is based on the ability to free hydrogen ions.

Very simply put, the pH scale measures the amount of oxygen in your blood. When your blood is too acid it will not carry enough oxygen. When it is too alkaline, it will carry too much.

The scale goes from 0 to 14. A pH of 7 is neutral, a pH of 0-7 is acid. A pH of 7-14 is alkaline. Each unit of change represents a tenfold change in acidity or alkalinity. Thus the difference between a pH of 4 and 5 is much greater than the difference between 6 an 7.

PH Scale

Thus your blood is in balance when you are slightly alkaline: a pH of 7.365.

How To Neutralize Harmful Acids

When you're just starting a raw food diet, it may be hard to become alkaline. Even if you eat raw greens all day. I find that juicing (with fruits or herbs for taste) speeds up this process tremendously, but it may still not be enough.

I that case, you may want to use some alkalizing supplements. Examples are (Himalayan) sea salt, pearl calcium, silica, pH drops, green powder, E3 Live or other super foods.

Summary

The list of alkaline food is all that's raw and green (especially greens, sea vegetables, superfoods and herbs) and an acid food list is all animal products, grains, sugars, fats and seeds. In order to stay alkaline 80% of your food should be alkaline and 20 acidic.

To test your pH you can buy pH test strips for less than $ 15,- (online, health store or pharmacy). The test will take 2 seconds.

Raw Food Diet Conversion Chart

Food

	Bad	Better	Best
Sugar	All forms: - Dextrose - Corn syrup - Rice syrup - Malt	Raw honey Raw Agave Maple syrup Raw fresh fruits Raisins Dates	Stevia Vanilla Cinnamon Raw honey (25g) and Coconut Sugar Raw fruit in moderation
Sweeteners	All forms: - Aspartame - Splenda	- Xylitol	Stevia Vanilla Cinnamon
Salt	Table salt Iodized salt	Unrefined sea salt Unrefined Celtic sea salt	Organic salt from plants: Celery Seaweed Phytoplankton
Flour	White flours from: - Wheat - Corn - Rice, etc.	Organic whole flours from: - Spelt* - Kamut - Quinoa - Buckwheat - Millet - Brown rice* - Other non stored grains *stored grain	Sprouted grains Almond flour Coconut flour
Bread	From supermarket	Home made Health store Sourdough (Yeast free) Wheat free Sprouted	Dehydrated flax crackers Essence bread Lettuce wraps

Pasta	White pasta	Organic spelt or buckwheat Sprouted pasta	(Raw) spaghetti made from squash
Fat	Butter Shortening Margarine Chemicals Trans fats Animal fats Fermented fats	Cold pressed coconut oil Olive oil Hemp seed oil Flax seed oil	Whole hemp seeds Whole organic flax Seeds Nuts Fresh coconut
Meat	Cold cuts Processed meat: Hot dogs Bacon Salami, etc.	Organic raised Nitrites free E-numbers free (EU) MSG free, etc.	Vegan nut pate's Raw "meat" balls made from nuts/seeds
Fish	Farm raised fish	Wild fish Not endangered	Wild Alaskan fish Caught same day & sustainable Cold smoked wild Alaskan salmon Krill Oil
Eggs	Conventional eggs	Organic farm free eggs	Egg replacers: - Agar agar - Flax seed - Psyllium fiber
Cheese	Cheese From cow Pasteurized Not organic Homogenized	Organic raw goat cheese Organic raw sheep's cheese	Nut cheese Seed cheese
Milk & Yogurt	Milk, yogurt From cow Pasteurized Homogenized	Organic milk Raw goat's milk Almond milk from store Rice milk Coconut milk	Raw almond milk Raw milk from nuts Raw milk from seeds & grains Home made Kefir Raw coconut juice & milk

Beverages

	Bad	Better	Best
Water	Water from tap	Plastic bottled water Evian, Poland Spring, Fuji Water	Distilled water Low mineral spring water Bottled in glass
Thee	Black tea		Herbal teas
Coffee	Coffee Decaffeinated coffee	Coffee replacer	Raw "hot" chocolate milk
Soft Drinks	Lemonade Jam Soft drinks Fruit juices	Organic fresh juices Flash pasteurized	Freshly squeezed juice: Fruit juice Orange Juice Vegetable juices Green powder juice Juice fresh from juice bar super foods drinks Coconut water (fresh) Smoothies Home made lemonade w stevia

Condiments And Spreads

	Bad	Better	Best
Tomato Ketchup	Tomato ketchup From supermarket	Organic, sugar free ketchup Home made ketchup	Raw ketchup
Mayonnaise	From super marked	Organic, no sugar added Home made	Raw home made mayonnaise Raw mayonnaise made from avocado Raw mayonnaise made from nuts/seeds
Pasta Sauces	From package Cans Mac n cheese Ready made	From health food store Organic Home made Pesto sauce Tomato sauce Organic Cheeses	Fresh raw tomato sauce Raw pesto Nut cheese Salsa
Bread Spreads	Cold cuts Processed meat Jam Chocolate spreads Cheese	Organic almond butter Jam/Jelly 100% fruit Raw honey Raw cheese	Avocado Pesto Tapenade Salsa Guacamole Nut pates Nut cheeses Coconut butter

Special Treats

	Bad	Better	Best
Candy	Candy from supermarket Energy bars Diet bars Chips Cookies	Organic from health store: - Candy - Chips - Cookies - Popcorn	Larabars Raw Cookies Raw cakes Fresh fruits Dried fruits Dehydrated crackers/ chips
Cookies, Cakes	Cookies from super marked Cakes from super marked	Organic from health store Home made cookies Home made cakes	Raw cookies & cakes Raw cakes & pies Dehydrated cookies

Supplements

	Bad	Better	Best
Supplements Vitamins	Supplements Vitamins From supermarket From drugstore	Supplements from some small companies	Whole foods supplements Super foods Green powders

General Food Guidelines

	Bad	Better	Best
Resources	Grocery store	Health store	Home made foods Green/farmer's market
Grown	Conventional grown	Organic foods Naturally grown No pesticides, herbicides, chemicals Local farmer's/ green market	Wild Local and organic Own garden, sprouts
Processed	Junk Pre-packaged Fast food Grilled Microwaved BBQ Fried	Steamed Cooked Stir fried Baked at low temperatures	Raw Juiced Blended Dehydrated
Ingredients	Many ingredients Conservatives Sweeteners Chemicals E-numbers MSG, flavor enhancers, etc.	Few ingredients Ingredients you can pronounce	Home made All fresh ingredients

CPSIA information can be obtained
at www.ICGtesting.com
Printed in the USA
LVHW011632160621
690393LV00009B/1119

9 781801 322355